Copyright © 2022 by Monica Dimitrios

Table of Contents

Fiber is the part of fruits, vegetables and grains not digested by your body. A low-fiber diet restricts these foods. As a result, the amount of undigested material passing through your large intestine is limited and stool bulk is lessened.

A low-fiber diet may be recommended for a number of conditions or situations. It is sometimes called a restricted-fiber diett.

LOW FIBER RECIPES

1. Fresh Mozzarella Strawberry Kale Salad

Prep Time: 15 mins

Total Time: 15 mins

Servings: 4

Ingredients

- 2 teaspoons agave nectar
- 1 tablespoon white wine vinegar
- ½ tablespoon extra-virgin olive oil
- 2 cups kale, chopped
- 5 large strawberries, sliced
- 2 tablespoons pine nuts
- ¼ cup chopped walnuts
- 2 ounces BelGioioso Fresh Mozzarella Pearls cheese

Directions

1. In a small bowl, whisk together agave, vinegar and olive oil. Add to kale and mix until leaves are coated.

2. Transfer to a bowl and top with strawberries, pine nuts, walnuts and Fresh Mozzarella.

2. Burrata Chicken Sliders

Prep Time: 20 mins

Total Time: 30 mins

Servings: 12

Ingredients

- 6 thinly sliced boneless chicken breasts
- 1 pinch Salt and pepper
- 1 tablespoon olive oil
- 12 slider buns, split
- 1 tomato, thinly sliced
- 12 fresh basil leaves
- 1 (8 ounce) package BelGioioso burrata cheese, sliced to include filling

Directions

1. Cut chicken breasts in half to fit a slider bun. Season both sides of chicken with salt and pepper. Lightly oil a grill or pan-grill over medium heat. Grill chicken until no longer pink inside, about 5 minutes per side. Set aside.

2. Toast buns by grilling them cut-side down. For each sandwich, layer cooked chicken breast, tomato slice, fresh basil leaf, and burrata slice between the toasted slider buns.

Prep Time: 30 mins

Total Time: 2 hrs 15 mins

Servings: 6

Ingredients

- 2 small eggplants, sliced
- 1 pinch Salt
- 4 tablespoons corn oil
- 2 tablespoons extra-virgin olive oil
- 2 cloves garlic, minced
- ¼ cup onions, chopped
- 4 large fresh tomatoes, chopped
- ¼ cup Fresh basil, chopped
- 4 ounces BelGioioso Ricotta con Latte® cheese
- 1 tablespoon heavy whipping cream
- 1 egg
- 8 ounces BelGioioso Fresh Mozzarella cheese, sliced

Directions

1. Arrange eggplant slices on paper towel and sprinkle with salt to weep out moisture; let sit for 1 hour. Heat corn oil in a deep saucepan and fry eggplant slices in the hot oil until tender. Drain oil.

2. Heat olive oil in large saucepan, add minced garlic and onions and saute. Add chopped tomatoes and stir. Simmer for 15 minutes and add fresh basil; set sauce aside.

3. Preheat oven to 325 degrees F. Combine Ricotta con Latte with cream, grated Parmesan, and egg to make a sauce; set aside.

4. Spread 1/2 cup of sauce in the bottom of a gratin dish and layer with the fried eggplant slices, Fresh Mozzarella, Ricotta mixture, and tomato sauce, until ingredients are used. Place in oven and bake until warm and slightly browned, 25 to 35 minutes. Garnish with grated Parmesan before serving.

4. Parmesan Crisp Salad

Prep Time: 15 mins

Total Time: 30 mins

Servings: 4

Ingredients

- 8 ounces BelGioioso Parmesan cheese, shredded
- 1 tablespoon white wine vinegar
- 3 tablespoons extra-virgin olive oil
- 2 cups Brussels sprouts, chopped
- 1 large orange, cut into wedges
- 2 tablespoons roasted hazelnuts, chopped
- ½ cup red grapes, halved

Directions

1. Preheat the oven to 350 degrees F (175 degrees C). Oil a sheet pan and place 1 tablespoon of shredded Parmesan in piles on the pan.
2. Bake for 8 minutes or until cheese starts to brown. Remove from oven and let cool for 1

minute. Remove crisps from the pan and cool completely.

3. In a small bowl, whisk together vinegar and olive oil. Add dressing to the chopped Brussels sprouts and toss until coated.

4. Transfer to serving bowl and top with orange wedges, hazelnuts, and red grapes. Garnish with Parmesan crisps.

5. Cannoli Cream with Cookies

Prep Time: 5 mins

Total Time: 35 mins

Servings: 6

Ingredients

- 1 (16 ounce) container BelGioioso Ricotta Con Latte
- ¼ cup white sugar
- 2 tablespoons semisweet chocolate chips
- 12 lemon-flavored shortbread cookies
- 6 mint sprigs

Directions

1. Combine BelGioioso Ricotta con Latte cheese with sugar until well blended. More sugar may be added if a sweeter filling is preferred. Stir in the chocolate chips; cover and refrigerate mixture for at least 30 minutes before serving.
2. To serve, scoop a serving of the cannoli cream onto a dessert plate and garnish with cookies and a mint sprig.

Prep Time: 15 mins

Total Time: 25 mins

Servings: 8

Ingredients

- 3 tablespoons extra-virgin olive oil
- 1 (10 ounce) package refrigerated pizza crust
- 4 ounces BelGioioso Mascarpone cheese
- 6 ounces BelGioioso CreamyGorg or Crumbly Gorgonzola cheese, thinly sliced
- 4 ounces BelGioioso Fresh Mozzarella cheese, sliced
- ¼ cup balsamic cipolline onions, sliced

Directions

1. Preheat oven to 400 degrees F. Coat a pizza pan with oil and spread the pizza dough evenly to all edges of the pizza pan. Spread BelGioioso Mascarpone over the pizza dough. Top with slices of BelGioioso Gorgonzola and Fresh Mozzarella

and cipolline onions. Bake for 10-15 minutes, until crust is golden brown and cheese is melted.

7. Glazed Pearl Onions with Raisins and Almonds

Servings: 8

Ingredients

- 2 pounds pearl onions
- 1 cup dry sherry
- ½ cup raisins
- ¼ cup honey
- ¼ cup water
- 2 tablespoons butter
- 1 teaspoon chopped fresh thyme
- ⅔ cup toasted slivered almonds
- 4 teaspoons red wine vinegar
- salt to taste
- ground black pepper to taste

Directions

1. Bring a pot of salted water to a boil. Add onions, and cook 3 minutes to loosen skins. Drain, and cool slightly. Cut root ends from onions.
2. Combine pearl onions, sherry, raisins, honey, water, butter or margarine, and thyme in a heavy large skillet. Bring to a boil over medium-high

heat. Reduce heat to very low, and cover. Simmer until liquid evaporates and onions begin to caramelize, stirring often, about 45 minutes. Season with salt and pepper. Remove from heat. Can be prepared 6 hours ahead. Let stand at room temperature. Rewarm over low heat before continuing.

3. Stir almonds and vinegar into onions. Add a few teaspoons of water if mixture is too dry. Serve warm.

8. Burrata Roasted Vegetable Pasta

Prep Time: 30 mins

Total Time: 50 mins

Servings: 10

Ingredients

- 1 cup balsamic vinegar
- 16 ounces fresh asparagus, trimmed
- 8 ounces button mushrooms, quartered
- 16 ounces Roma tomatoes, quartered
- 16 ounces small zucchini squash, sliced thinly lengthwise
- 1 small bunch Italian parsley, chopped
- 1 cup extra virgin olive oil
- 3 cloves garlic, crushed
- 2 tablespoons kosher salt
- 2 tablespoons cracked black pepper
- 1 (16 ounce) package gemelli pasta
- 1 leaf Fresh basil leaves, torn into small pieces
- 8 ounces BelGioioso burrata cheese, sliced

Directions

1. Preheat oven to 425 degrees F. In a large saucepan over high heat, boil balsamic vinegar until it is reduced to half. Remove from heat and let cool.

2. In a large bowl, combine asparagus, mushrooms, tomatoes, zucchini, parsley, olive oil, garlic, salt and pepper. Toss to incorporate olive oil. Place vegetables onto a large sheet pan and bake for 10-12 minutes, stirring halfway through.

3. Meanwhile, fill a large pot with lightly salted water and bring to a rolling boil. Stir in pasta and return to a boil. Cook pasta uncovered, stirring occasionally, until tender yet firm to the bite, 12 to 13 minutes.

4. Remove vegetables from oven and let cool. Drizzle with reduced balsamic to taste. Add more salt and pepper if desired.

5. Toss cooked pasta with fresh basil and olive oil and place into serving bowls. Top with roasted vegetable mixture. Place sliced Burrata on top of

vegetables, drizzle with olive oil, and garnish with fresh basil.

9. Wild Mushroom and Pea Pasta

Prep Time: 20 mins

Total Time: 40 mins

Servings: 4

Ingredients

- 1 (16 ounce) package orecchiette pasta
- 2 tablespoons unsalted butter
- 3 cups assorted wild mushrooms, cleaned and sliced
- 4 each Roma tomatoes, diced
- 2 cups frozen green peas
- ½ cup heavy whipping cream
- 4 ounces BelGioioso Mascarpone cheese
- 1 cup BelGioioso Parmesan cheese, grated
- 16 ounces BelGioioso Fresh Mozzarella cheese
- 1 pinch Kosher salt
- ¼ teaspoon Black pepper

Directions

1. Fill a large pot with lightly salted water and bring to a rolling boil. Stir in pasta and return to a boil. Cook pasta uncovered, stirring occasionally, until tender yet firm to the bite, 9 to 12 minutes. Drain and let cool.

2. In a large pan, heat butter over medium-high heat. Add sliced wild mushrooms and saute for 1 minute. Stir in Roma tomatoes and peas. Add heavy cream, Mascarpone, Parmesan, and Fresh Mozzarella. Stir to combine.

3. Toss pasta into the sauce and season with salt and pepper to taste. Serve immediately.

10. Brandied Pears with Mascarpone Cream Sauce

Prep Time: 10 mins

Total Time: 20 mins

Servings: 8

Ingredients

- 4 large fresh pears, each sliced into 6 wedges
- 1 lemon, juiced
- 2 tablespoons unsalted butter
- ½ cup brown sugar
- ¼ cup brandy
- 8 ounces BelGioioso Mascarpone cheese
- ¼ cup pure maple syrup

Directions

1. Toss pear slices in lemon juice to prevent browning. Melt butter in large pan over low heat. Add sliced pears and saute for a few minutes until heated through. Add brown sugar and stir until melted and the pears are coated. Heat mixture until pears start to soften, then add brandy.

2. Bring to a boil and poach pears until soft and heated through.

3. Mix mascarpone with maple syrup and serve pears warm or slightly cooled with a dollop of mascarpone cream sauce.

11. Fresh Mozzarella Tortellini Skewers

Prep Time: 15 mins

Total Time: 23 mins

Servings: 8

Ingredients

8 ounces mini tortellini pasta

- 8 ounces BelGioioso Fresh Mozzarella cheese
- 1 leaf Fresh basil leaves
- 12 Grape tomatoes
- 8 wooden skewers
- 2 tablespoons Pesto dipping sauce, prepared

Directions

1. Fill a large pot with lightly salted water and bring to a rolling boil; stir in tortellini and return to a boil. Cook uncovered, stirring occasionally, until the tortellini float to the top and the filling is hot, about 3 minutes. Let cool completely.

2. If necessary, cut fresh mozzarella into 1-inch pieces. Thread Fresh Mozzarella, fresh basil

leaves, tortellini and tomatoes onto skewers. Serve with prepared pesto as a dipping sauce.

12. Lasagna Noodle Soup

Prep Time: 20 mins

Total Time: 45 mins

Servings: 8

Ingredients

- 1 pound lean ground beef
- 1 cup diced onion
- 3 cloves garlic, minced
- 2 (14.5 ounce) cans diced tomatoes
- 1 (8 ounce) can tomato sauce
- ¼ cup tomato paste
- 4 cups low-sodium beef broth
- 2 teaspoons Italian seasoning
- 6 each uncooked lasagna noodles, broken into 1/2-inch pieces
- 1 pinch Salt and pepper
- 8 ounces BelGioioso Ricotta Con Latte
- ½ cup BelGioioso Grated Parmesan cheese

Directions

1. In a large saucepan, brown beef and onion over medium-high heat, 5 to 7 minutes. Add the garlic and cook for 30 to 60 seconds. Drain.

2. Stir in diced tomatoes, tomato saucc, tomato paste, beef broth, and Italian seasoning. Bring mixture to a boil and stir in lasagna noodles. Reduce heat slightly and cook for 10 minutes, or until noodles are tender. Season with salt and pepper to taste.

3. For the cheese topping, in a small bowl, mix together the Ricotta and Parmesan.

4. To serve, spoon soup into a bowl and top with a spoonful of the cheese mixture.

13. Butternut-Yogurt Bread

Prep Time: 15 mins

Total Time: 1 hr 50 mins

Servings: 6

Ingredients

- 1 butternut squash, unpeeled
- ¾ cup white whole wheat flour
- ⅓ cup shredded part-skim mozzarella cheese
- ½ teaspoon baking soda
- ¼ teaspoon baking powder
- ¼ teaspoon ground coriander
- 1 egg
- ¼ cup fat-free Greek yogurt
- 2 tablespoons unsweetened applesauce
- 1 tablespoon cold-pressed olive oil
- 2 tablespoons sunflower seeds

Directions

1. Preheat the oven to 350 degrees F (175 degrees C). Line a baking sheet with aluminum foil. Poke

holes all over the surface of the butternut squash using a fork. Place on the baking sheet.

2. Bake squash in the preheated oven until tender, about 50 minutes. Remove and let cool. Reduce oven temperature to 365 degrees F (185 degrees C).

3. Combine flour, mozzarella cheese, baking soda, baking powder, and coriander in a bowl.

4. Peel and cube butternut squash. Measure 1/2 cup into a blender; refrigerate the rest. Add egg, Greek yogurt, applesauce, and oil to the blender. Blend until bubbly, about 5 minutes. Pour into the bowl with the flour mixture and mix well. Spoon the thick batter into a 7 1/2-inch cast iron skillet. Sprinkle sunflower seeds on top.

5. Bake in the preheated oven until a toothpick inserted into the center comes out clean, about 40 minutes. Let cool for 5 minutes before slicing.

14. Kohlrabi and Pea Soup with Dill

Prep Time: 15 mins

Total Time: 45 mins

Servings: 2

Ingredients

- 1 tablespoon olive oil
- ½ large onion, chopped
- 1 pound peas
- ½ pound kohlrabi, peeled and cut into small dice
- 1 bunch fresh dill, chopped
- ½ tablespoon seasoning blend
- water to cover

Directions

1. Heat oil in a saucepan over medium heat. Add onion and cook until wilted, about 3 minutes. Add peas and kohlrabi; stir to combine. Add dill and seasoning blend; stir to combine.
2. Add water to cover vegetables and bring to a boil. Reduce heat and cover halfway with a lid. Cook

until peas and kohlrabi are soft, about 20 minutes more. Cool to room temperature before serving.

15. Boar's Head Bold Bourbon Ridge Uncured Smoked Ham Summer Salad

Prep Time: 20 mins

Total Time: 20 mins

Servings: 4

Ingredients

For the Dressing:

- ½ cup champagne vinegar
- 3 tablespoons Boar's Head Real Mayonnaise
- 1 green onion, white and green parts, minced
- 1 ½ teaspoons honey
- 2 teaspoons Dijon mustard
- 1 small garlic clove, minced
- 1 tablespoon fresh lemon juice
- 1 teaspoon chopped fresh dill
- 1 teaspoon chopped fresh parsley leaves
- 1 teaspoon kosher salt
- ½ teaspoon freshly ground black pepper
- 1 cup canola oil
- 2 ½ cups mixed salad greens

- 8 ounces Boar's Head Bold Bourbon Ridge Uncured Smoked Ham, sliced thin
- 1 cup peaches, sliced thin
- ½ cup blueberries
- ½ cup raspberries
- ½ cup blackberries

Directions

1. To make the dressing, combine the vinegar, mayonnaise, green onion, honey, Dijon mustard, garlic, lemon juice, dill, parsley, salt, and pepper in a blender or food processor with a metal blade. With the machine running, gradually add the oil in a thin, steady stream to form an emulsion. Set aside when complete.
2. Place mixed greens into a large salad bowl, top with dressing and remaining ingredients, and serve.

16. Shredded Broccoli Salad

Prep Time: 5 mins

Total Time: 5 mins

Servings: 6

Ingredients

- 1 (10 ounce) package shredded broccoli slaw
- 1 cup crumbled feta cheese
- 1 cup Italian-style salad dressing
- ½ cup raisins
- ½ cup sweetened dried cranberries

Directions

1. Mix broccoli slaw, feta cheese, salad dressing, raisins, and dried cranberries together in a large bowl. Toss with a fork or cover with a lid and shake.

Prep Time: 15 mins

Total Time: 4 hrs 15 mins

Servings: 6

Ingredients

- 2 (10 ounce) packages frozen peas, defrosted
- ½ cup fresh lime juice
- 2 cups plain yogurt
- ½ cup olive oil
- 4 cloves garlic, smashed
- 1 tablespoon chili powder
- 2 cups ice water
- 2 tablespoons kosher salt
- ¼ cup red bell pepper, chopped, or more to taste
- 2 tablespoons chopped tomatoes, or to taste
- 1 tablespoon chopped jalapeno pepper, or to taste

Directions

1. Puree peas in a food processor or blender, constantly scraping down the sides. If peas are too dry, add a little of the lime juice.

2. Add remaining lime juice, yogurt, olive oil, garlic, and chili powder. Blend until liquefied. Pour into a large bowl; add ice water and salt and stir to incorporate. Refrigerate until flavors combine, at least 4 to 6 hours.

3. Garnish each serving with red pepper, tomato, and jalapeno.

18. Sarah's Quick Warm Lentil Salad

Prep Time: 5 mins

Total Time: 40 mins

Servings: 4

Ingredients

- 1 cup dry lentils
- 1 cup chicken broth
- water to cover
- 2 tablespoons unsalted butter
- 1 medium onion, chopped
- 1 teaspoon minced garlic
- 1 (14 ounce) can diced tomatoes, drained
- 1 teaspoon salt
- 1 tablespoon balsamic vinegar

Directions

1. Combine lentils and chicken broth in a pot. Add just enough water to cover. Bring to a low simmer and cook until lentils are cooked, but not falling

apart, about 25 minutes. Add water when necessary in order to keep lentils covered.

2. Melt butter in a saucepan over medium heat and cook onion until translucent and slightly browned, about 5 minutes. Add garlic and saute for 30 seconds. Add lentils and their liquid to the saucepan. Gently fold in tomatoes. Season with salt, add in balsamic vinegar, and stir gently. Serve warm.

19. Chicken Florentine Dip

Prep Time: 15 mins

Total Time: 1 hr 45 mins

Servings: 10

Ingredients

- 2 (10.5 ounce) cans condensed, 98% fat-free cream of chicken soup with 30% less sodium
- 9 ounces diced cooked chicken
- 1 (8 ounce) container reduced-fat sour cream
- 2 cups shredded part-skim mozzarella cheese
- ½ cup skim milk, or more as needed
- ½ cup grated Parmesan cheese
- 1 (10 ounce) package frozen chopped spinach - thawed, drained, and squeezed dry

Directions

1. Combine condensed soup, chicken, sour cream mozzarella cheese, 1/2 cup skim milk, and Parmesan cheese in a slow cooker. Add spinach,

pulling it apart and shredding it as you put it in. Mix until well blended.

2. Cover and cook on Low until all cheeses are melted and the dip is deliciously gooey, 1 to 1 1/2 hours. Add up to 1/2 cup more milk if you feel the dip is cooking up too thick.

20. Grandma Knobel's Crepes

Prep Time: 10 mins

Total Time: 25 mins

Servings: 3

Ingredients

- 1 cup all-purpose flour
- ½ cup white sugar
- ¼ teaspoon salt
- 1 ½ cups milk
- 3 large eggs
- ½ teaspoon vanilla extract
- 1 tablespoon avocado oil, divided, or as needed
- 1 tablespoon unsalted butter, or to taste
- 2 tablespoons maple syrup, or to taste
- 1 tablespoon powdered sugar, or to taste

Directions

1. Sift flour, sugar, and salt into a large bowl. Add milk, eggs, and vanilla and whisk until smooth and slightly thinner than a regular pancake

batter; do not overmix the batter or it will result in tougher crepes.

2. Heat an 8- to 10-inch skillet over medium heat. Add 1 teaspoon oil to the center of the pan.

3. Pour about 1/2 cup batter into the dot of oil. Hold the skillet by the handle and tilt the pan around so the batter evenly coats the entire skillet; the crepe should be about 1/8-inch thick. Cook until the bottom is medium brown, the top is dry, and the edges are starting to curl, about 1 minute. Flip the crepe and cook until golden brown on the other side, about 30 seconds. If each crepe takes longer than 2 minutes to cook, the batter may need to be thinner or you may need to use a higher heat.

4. Place crepe on a plate with a dab of butter on top. Drizzle with maple syrup, roll up, dust with powdered sugar, and serve.

5. Repeat Steps 3 and 4, adding more avocado oil to the skillet as needed.

21. Citrus Honey Brined Smoked Turkey

Prep Time: 30 mins

Total Time: 12 hrs 30 mins

Servings: 20

Ingredients

- 1 gallon hot water
- 1 pound kosher salt
- 2 quarts vegetable broth
- 2 (8 ounce) jars honey
- 1 cup orange juice
- 1 (7 pound) bag of ice cubes
- 1 (15 pound) whole turkey, neck and giblets removed
- ¼ cup vegetable oil
- 1 teaspoon poultry seasoning
- 1 Granny Smith apple, cored and cut into large chunks
- 1 stalk celery, cut into chunks
- 1 small onion, cut into chunks
- 1 orange, quartered

Directions

1. Mix hot water and kosher salt in a 54-quart cooler, stirring until the salt dissolves. Mix in vegetable broth, honey, and orange juice. Pour in the ice cubes, place the turkey into the brine with breast side up, and close the cooler lid. Place the cooler in a cold place and let the turkey marinate overnight or up to 12 hours. Brine temperature must stay colder than 40 degrees F (4 degrees C).

2. Remove turkey from brine, discard brine, and dry the turkey thoroughly with paper towels. Mix vegetable oil with poultry seasoning in a bowl, and rub the turkey with the mixture. Place apple, celery, onion, and orange pieces into the cavity of the turkey.

3. Preheat an outdoor grill to 400 degrees F (205 degrees C) for indirect heat and lightly oil the grate. Build a 'smoke bomb' by placing about 1 cup of hickory or cherry wood chips into the middle of a 12x12-inch doubled piece of aluminum foil. Gather up the edges of the foil to make a pouch and leave the pouch open at the

top. Set the smoke bomb directly onto the coals if grilling with charcoal, or onto the flame bar of a gas grill.

4. Set the turkey onto the grill in position for indirect heat, insert a probe thermometer into the thickest part of the turkey breast, not touching a bone, and close the grill. Set the probe thermometer for 160 degrees F (70 degrees C).

5. Grill turkey for 1 hour and check the bird; if skin is already golden brown, cover the breast, legs, and wings with aluminum foil. Replace the smoke bomb with a new one; close cover and continue to grill until probe thermometer registers 160 degrees F (70 degrees C), 2 to 3 more hours. Remove the fruit and vegetable pieces from the cavity, cover turkey with aluminum foil, and let rest for 1 hour before carving.

22. Funfetti Style Cookies

Prep Time: 10 mins

Total Time: 19 mins

Servings: 48

Ingredients

- 1 cup butter, softened
- 1 cup sour cream
- 1 cup white sugar
- 2 eggs
- ½ cup multicolored candy sprinkles
- ½ cup confectioners' sugar
- 1 tablespoon cornstarch, or more as needed
- 1 ½ teaspoons vanilla extract
- 1 teaspoon almond extract
- 1 teaspoon baking powder
- ½ teaspoon baking soda
- ½ teaspoon salt
- ½ teaspoon nutmeg
- ½ teaspoon ground cinnamon
- 2 cups all-purpose flour, or more as needed

Directions

1. Preheat oven to 325 degrees F (165 degrees C). Line 2 baking sheets with parchment paper.

2. Beat butter, sour cream, white sugar, and eggs together in a large bowl with an electric mixer until light and fluffy. Beat in candy sprinkles, confectioners' sugar, cornstarch, vanilla extract, almond extract, baking powder, baking soda, salt, nutmeg, and cinnamon until fully incorporated, 1 to 2 minutes. Beat flour in gradually until sticky dough forms, 1 to 2 minutes more. Drop spoonfuls of dough 2 inches apart onto prepared baking sheets.

3. Bake in the preheated oven until edges are golden, 9 to 13 minutes. Cool on the baking sheet for 1 minute before removing to a wire rack to cool completely.

23. Light Rose Water Lemonade

Prep Time: 5 mins

Total Time: 5 mins

Servings: 4

Ingredients

- 4 cups water
- 1 cup freshly squeezed lemon juice
- ⅓ cup granulated sugar substitute
- ⅓ cup rose water
- 1 pinch salt
- ice

Directions

1. Combine water, lemon juice, sugar substitute, rose water, and salt in a large pitcher; stir well.
2. Chill lemonade in the refrigerator. Serve over ice.

Prep Time: 5 mins

Total Time: 1 hr 25 mins

Servings: 10

Ingredients

- 2 tablespoons quick-cooking oats
- 1 cup milk
- ½ cup water
- 2 large eggs
- 1 tablespoon butter, melted
- 1 teaspoon white sugar
- ¼ teaspoon salt
- ½ cup all-purpose flour
- ½ cup whole wheat flour

Directions

1. Place oats in a blender and blend on high speed to make oat flour, 10 to 15 seconds. Add milk, water, eggs, melted butter, sugar, and salt and blend

until combined. Add both flours and blend until incorporated and smooth, about 20 seconds.

2. Refrigerate batter for 1 hour.

3. Remove batter from the refrigerator and blend for a few seconds if batter has separated.

4. Heat a 12-inch saucepan over medium heat. Spray the warm pan with nonstick spray. Add 1/4 cup batter to the pan, lifting and swirling the pan immediately so the batter spreads thinly and uniformly around the pan. Cook until the edges are set and begin to pull away from the pan, 1 to 3 minutes. Flip crepe with a rubber spatula and cook for another 30 seconds. Remove to a cooling rack and repeat to cook remaining crepes.

25. Stuffed Salsa Verde Potatoes with Leftover Turkey

Prep Time: 15 mins

Total Time: 1 hr 30 mins

Servings: 4

Ingredients

- 4 medium potatoes
- ¾ cup shredded or cubed cooked turkey
- ¾ cup green salsa
- 1 lightly packed fresh cilantro leaves and tender stems ½ cup sour cream, or more to taste
- 2 tablespoons cream cheese, softened
- 2 tablespoons butter, softened
- salt and ground black pepper to taste
- 4 tablespoons shredded Mexican cheese blend, or to taste

Directions

1. Preheat an oven to 450 degrees F (230 degrees C). Prick potatoes several times with a fork and place onto a baking sheet.

2. Bake in the preheated oven until potatoes are easily pierced with a fork, 50 minutes to 1 hour. Remove from the oven and allow to cool slightly; leave oven on.

3. Mix turkey, salsa, and chile pepper together in a bowl.

4. Make a slice in the top of each potato and scoop out the inside. Place in a bowl and mash. Add turkey-salsa mixture, sour cream, cream cheese, butter, salt, and pepper; mix to desired consistency. Fill potatoes with mixture and sprinkle Mexican cheese on top.

5. Return to the oven and bake until heated through, about 15 minutes.

Prep Time: 15 mins

Total Time: 45 mins

Servings: 10

Ingredients

- 1 ½ cups fresh pumpkin seeds, washed and dried
- ¼ cup brown sugar
- 1 tablespoon ground cinnamon
- 1 tablespoon curry powder
- 3 tablespoons vegetable oil, or as needed

Directions

1. Preheat oven to 325 degrees F (165 degrees C).
2. Combine pumpkin seeds, brown sugar, cinnamon, and curry powder in a bowl. Add vegetable oil gradually, until lightly coated. Spread seeds evenly on a baking sheet.
3. Bake in the preheated oven for 10 minutes. Remove the sheet from the oven and flip the seeds. Continue baking, flipping seeds every 10

minutes, until crunchy and golden brown, 20 to 30 minutes.

27. Soy Chorizo Taco Filling

Prep Time: 15 mins

Total Time: 30 mins

Servings: 12

Ingredients

- 2 tablespoons vegetable oil
- 8 ounces soy chorizo, cut into bite-sized pieces
- 2 green bell peppers, cut into bite-sized pieces
- 1 red bell peppers, cut into bite-sized pieces
- 1 medium onion, cut into bite-sized pieces
- ½ cup water
- 1 tablespoon taco seasoning mix, or to taste
- 1 teaspoon hot sauce, or to taste
- 1 teaspoon paprika, or more to taste

Directions

1. Heat oil in a skillet over medium-high heat. Add chorizo and cook until slightly browned, about 5 minutes. Add bell peppers and onion and cook until slightly soft but still firm, about 5 minutes

more. Add water and taco seasoning. Stir until thoroughly mixed and water is bubbly. Reduce heat to medium and let water reduce, 3 to 4 minutes. Add hot sauce and paprika.

Prep Time: 15 mins

Total Time: 17 mins

Servings: 10

Ingredients

- 1 (14 ounce) package chocolate sandwich cookies
- 12 ounces red candy melts
- multicolored sprinkles (jimmies)

Directions

1. Place candy melts in a microwave-safe bowl. Microwave for 1 minute. Stir. Microwave for 30 seconds more. Stir. Repeat process until candy melts are completely liquid.
2. Dip sandwich cookies into the melted candy melts - feel free to coat only half of the cookie, or coat all sides. Place red cookies on a plate lined with wax paper.
3. Decorate with assorted sprinkles. Allow to harden before removing to serve.

29. Spicy Cocoa Almonds

Prep Time: 5 mins

Total Time: 20 mins

Servings: 16

Ingredients

- 4 cups raw unsalted almonds
- 2 tablespoons unsweetened cocoa powder
- 1 teaspoon granular sucralose sweetener
- 1 teaspoon cayenne pepper

Directions

1. Preheat the oven to 350 degrees F (175 degrees C). Place the almonds in a single layer on a rimmed baking tray.
2. Bake in the preheated oven for 5 minutes. Stir and continue baking until fragrant and toasty, about 5 minutes more. Let cool on tray for 2 minutes; pour into a bowl.
3. Add cocoa powder, sucralose, and cayenne pepper. Stir with a spatula until well coated. Pour

almonds back onto the baking tray to cool completely.

30. Chicken-Bacon Pressed Picnic Sandwiches

Prep Time: 15 mins

Total Time: 8 hrs 15 mins

Servings: 4

Ingredients

- ¼ cup raspberry preserves
- 3 tablespoons horseradish mustard, or to taste
- 1 (1 pound) loaf bread
- 6 ounces Louis Rich Deli Thin Rstd Chicken Breast
- 6 thick slices cooked bacon
- 2 slices Havarti cheese
- 4 leaves romaine lettuce, chopped

Directions

1. Combine raspberry preserves and horseradish mustard in a bowl and whisk or stir until evenly blended. Reserve a little sauce for serving.
2. Slice loaf of bread in half. Slather the bottom half generously with remaining sauce. Layer the

chicken, bacon, cheese (cut slices to fit as needed), and lettuce over the sauce layer, then top with remaining bread half.

3. Wrap sandwich in plastic wrap and place on a baking sheet. Place a second baking sheet on top and add books (or something that has some weight to it) to press the sandwich. Transfer to the refrigerator until flavors have melded, 8 hours to overnight.

4. When ready to serve, unwrap sandwich and slice into 4 pieces. Serve with additional sauce.

www.ingramcontent.com/pod-product-compliance
Lightning Source LLC
Chambersburg PA
CBHW070722260726
48660CB00007B/2687